Keto Dessert

Cookbook

The healthiest

keto dessert recipes

Sommario

INTRODUCTION

Welcome to the world of Keto sweets!

How can you stay in shape without rewarding yourself with good, juicy desserts?

In this book, I wanted to put my 50 favorite keto dessert recipes so you can wow your whole family and friends. Show off your fit physique while eating a delicious dessert.

Let's get started right away by baking these low-sugar protein desserts that are ideal for the whole family, so put on your apron and let's get started right away.

DESSERT RECIPES

412. <u>COCONUT CAKE</u>

Ingredients

- 2 cups unsalted butter bar

- 8 large eggs

- 1 ½ cups sucralose sweetener (sugar substitute)

- 3 tsp coconut extract

- 2/3 cup whole wheat flour

- 1 tsp baking powder (straight phosphate, double effect)

- ¼ tsp salt

- 6 large Protein

- 2/3 cup dried coconut

Instructions

1. Heat oven to 350° F. Grease 2 8-inch cake pans; line bottoms with parchment paper; Then grease the paper. Melt ½ cup butter and set aside. Place the remaining butter (1 ½ cups) on a plate, cut into 1 Tbsp portions, and store at room temperature.

2. Beat eggs with a high power electric mixer, 3/4 cup sugar substitute and 1 Tbsp coconut extract until ribbons form, about 5 min

3. In 3 additions, filter the soy flour, boiling power, and salt over the egg mixture; fold with a spatula to combine.

4. Double ½ cup melted butter. Then for the dough into the prepared shapes.

5. Bake for 22 min. Let cool in pans on a wire rack for 5 min Cover the boards with paper towels and inverted cake layers. Carefully peel off the parchment and allow it to cool completely.

6. For the frosting: put in a double kettle or in a bowl over boiling water over low heat, beat the egg whites, 3/4 cup

sugar substitute and salt until the temperature reaches 130° F. Transfer the egg whites to a bowl and beat on high speed until it is cold and utterly vanquished. Reduce rate to medium and mix 1 ½ cups butter at room temperature 1 Tbsp at a time until well combined, thick and creamy, about 10 min;

7. Place a layer of cake on a serving platter. Mix 1 cup icing with half the coconut (⅓ cup), a lower layer oFrost. Place the top cake layer on the bottom layer. Cover the top and sides with the remaining frosting and pat the remaining ⅓ cup coconut on the coating. Optional: toast with coconut (3-5 min at 350° F).

Prep time: 30 min; **Servings:** 12

Macros: 4.7 g net Carbs 8.9 g protein 39 g fat 1.6 g fiber 402.6 Cal

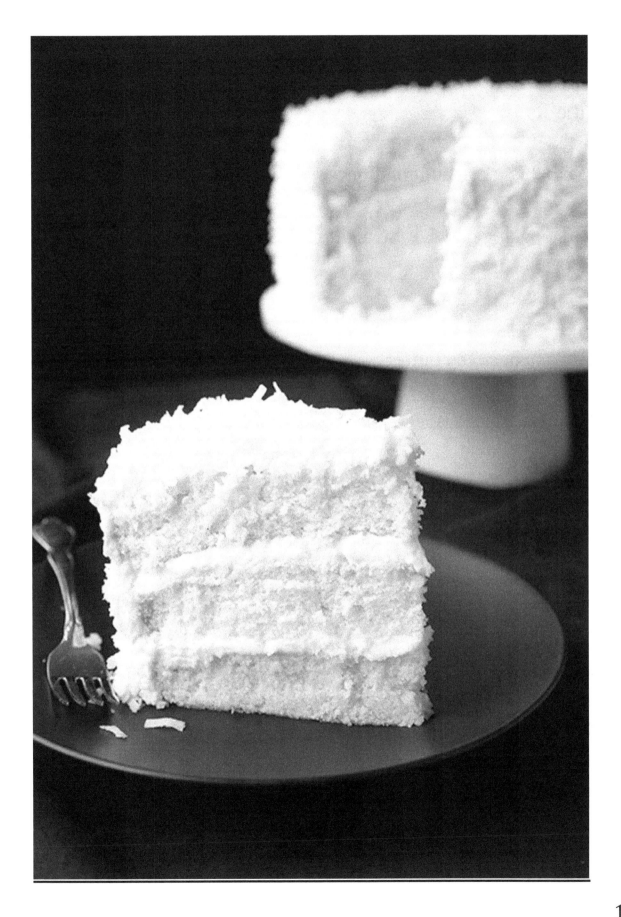

CARDAMOM BUTTER

Ingredients

- ½ cup blanched almond flour

- ¼ tsp baking powder (straight phosphate, double effect)

- ½ tsp salt

- 10 Tbsp unsalted butter

- ½ cup sucralose sweetener (sugar substitute)

- 1 large egg (whole)

- 1 Tbsp tap water

- 2 tsp vanilla extract

- 3/4 tsp ground cardamom

- 4 2/3 Servings:, flour mixture

Instructions

1. Use the flour mixture (or the gluten-free version) for this . To make 12 Servings:, you need 1 ½ cups of the mix. If you change the size of the portion to increase or decrease it, you must adjust it accordingly. Each serving of the baking blend represents ⅓ cup.

2. Preheat the oven to 350° F. Cover 2 baking sheets with parchment paper; put aside.

3. In a medium bowl, add 1 ½ cup baking mixture, ½ cup almond flour, baking powder, and salt. In a large bowl, blend butter and sugar substitute; cream until soft and fluffy with an electric mixer at high speed. Add the egg, sugar, vanilla, and cardamom; beat until smooth at medium speed; scrape the bowl sides if necessary (the mixture can appear watery). Add the flour mixture; blend until the dough is gathered.

4. Cut the dough in half and then again in half. Create 6 equal balls out of every quarter of the dough piece. Place on baking sheet 12 mixture. Gently squeeze each with the teeth of a grid fork (optional); cook about 10 min on the light brown edge. Or put it 30 min in the refrigerator and spread it over the

parchment; cut the shapes and cook. To cool them, move cookies to a wire rack. Store up to 1 week in an airtight container. Makes 2 cookies for each serving.

Prep time:10 min; **Servings:** 6

Macros: 3.5 g of net Carbs 8.8 g of protein 14 g oFat 1.7 g oFiber 176.6 of Cal

CHERRY COBBLER

Ingredients

- ¼ cup, half walnuts

- ½ cup sucralose sweetener (sugar substitute)

- 3/4 cinnamon tsp

- ¼ tsp salt

- 3 Tbsp unsalted butter bar

- ⅓ cup heavy cream

- 2 sour cream Tbsp (cultivated)

- 1 large egg (whole)

- 3 cups, no Sweet bites cherries

- ¼ tsp pure almond extract

- 2 ¼ Servings:, flour mixture

Instructions

1. For the cookies: Mix baking mix, nuts, 2 Tbsp sugar substitute, ½ tsp cinnamon, and salt in a food processor until it is moderately ground. Add the butter and squeeze until mixture looks like a full meal.

2. Beat the heavy cream, sour cream, and an egg in a cup or bowl to measure liquids. Pour into a food processor and press until everything is well mixed. Remove the dough and tap on a flat disc. Cover with plastic wrap and allow to cool for 1 to 2 hours.

3. For the filling: Preheat the oven to 400° F. Mix the cherries in a medium bowl with ⅓ cup sugar substitute, almond extract, and ¼ tsp cinnamon. Pour the filling into an 8-inch square or round baking dish. Divide the dough into 8 pieces and pat it on discs about 3 wide.

4. Alternate the cookies on the filling and bake for 35 to 40 min, until the cookies are golden and cooked and the fruit bubbles are soft. Serve with fresh whipped cream (optional).

Prep time:30 min; **Servings:** 8

Macros: 7.4 g protein 12.9 g fat 2.5 g fiber 191.2 Cal 11 g net Carbs

CHOCOLATE CHIP COOKIES

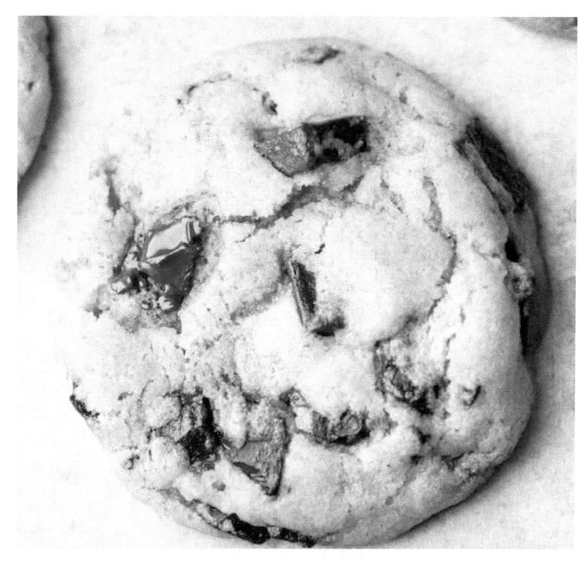

Ingredients

● 1 tsp baking powder

● ½ tsp salt

● 1 cup butter (salted)

- 1 cup sucralose sweetener (sugar substitute)

- 2 tsp vanilla extract

- 2 large eggs (whole)

- 4 g sugar-free Chocolate Chips

- 6 Servings:, flour mixture

Instructions

1. Preheat the oven to 375° F.

2. Combine all dry ingredients in a small bowl, set aside.

3. Mix melted butter, sugar substitute, and vanilla on medium speed with an electric mixer until everything is well combined. Add eggs 1 by 1 and mix well after each addition. Gradually add the mixture of dry ingredients and beat until well blended. Thoroughly mix the chocolate chips with a wooden spoon or spatula (4 oz or about 2/3 of a cup).

4. A spoon of rounded tsp cookie dough on a baking sheet covered with a spray of non-stick vegetable oil. Carefully

flatten the cookies by squeezing them with your hand or with a spatula.

5. Bake for 10 to 12 min or until light brown. Remove from the baking sheet and place cookies on a cooling rack.

Prep time: 20 min; **Servings:** 6

Macros: 2 g net Carbs 3.8 g protein 7.1 g fat 1.4 g fiber 86.7 Cal Cal

CHOCOLATE AND CLOUD MUFFINS

Ingredients

- 1-oz cream cheese

- 1 large egg

- 1 Tbsp vegetable oil

- 2 vanilla whey protein Tbsp

- 2 tsp cocoa powder (sugar-free)

- 2 tsp xylitol

- ¼ tsp baking powder (sodium and aluminum sulfate, double effect)

- ½ cinnamon tsp

- A pinch of salt

- 1 packet of 100% natural stevia sweetener

Instructions

1. Put the cream cheese in a microwave-safe cup. Heat for 10-15 seconds (enough to heat the cream cheese but not to melt it completely).

2. Add the egg and oil, mixing with the cream cheese.

3. Mix in a small bowl to combine the whey protein powder, cocoa powder, xylitol, baking powder, cinnamon, and a pinch of salt and stevia

4. Add the chocolate mixture to the cream cheese mixture in the cup; Stir to combine.

5. Heat the cup in the microwave for 1 minute.

Prep time:5 mins; **Servings:** 1

Macros: 2.9 g net Carbs 19.7 g protein 29 g fat 1.8 g fiber 370.7 Cal

FROZEN CHOCOLATE PUDDING POPS

Ingredients

- 1 each, generous dark chocolate smoothie

- 3/4 cup heavy cream, liquid

- 1 Tbsp cocoa powder

- 1 Tbsp erythritol

- ¼ tsp xanthan gum

Instructions

1. You need silicone molds for this .

2. Put all the ingredients in a high power mixer and mix about half at maximum speed for about 2 min The mixture should be a little frothy and well combined.

3. Pour mixture into silicone molds and place in the freezer until it is firm, according to the instructions of the silicone mold. Use within 2 weeks oFreezing.

Prep time:5 min; **Servings:** 1

Macros: 2 g net Carbs 4.9 g protein 18.9 g fat 1.5 g fiber 196.9 Cal

CHOCOLATE MACAROON AND GANACHE

Ingredients

- 3 large Protein

- 1 tsp fresh lemon juice

- 2 Tbsp xylitol

- 3/4 cup almond flour

- 6 Tbsp Sugar-Free Chocolate Chips

- 2 Tbsp heavy cream

Instructions

8. First, measure xylitol in the form of granules for this , then sprinkle it in a blender.

9. Preheat the oven to 250 ° F. Prepare a parchment paper on a baking sheet. It may be helpful to draw 1-inch circles on the back of the parchment. Put aside.

10. Beat the egg whites, lemon juice, a pinch of salt, and 1 Tbsp (x 3 tsp) of xylitol in a hard spot using an accessory whisk.

11. Sift the remaining Tbsp xylitol and almond flour together. Add to protein and fold gently to incorporate. Use a pastry bag or simply cut off the end of a large plastic bag with zipper, fill it with meringue and place it on the baking sheet and make 1-inch circles. If there are still spikes, touch the top with a slightly damp finger. Cook 35 to 45 min If they turn brown, lower the temperature by 25 F and cook a little more. Remove from the oven and let cool. Once cool, remove it with a spatula and place it on a piece of parchment paper.

12. Fill the filling: melt the chocolate in the microwave at 30-second intervals. Add the heavy cream and use a hand blender; Beat until thickened. Place the chocolate with an envelope sachet on the flat side of 1 macaroni and cover on the other side on the other flat side. Sprinkle with cocoa powder as a garnish if desired.

Prep time: 15 min

Macros: 1.1 g net Carbs 1.8 g protein 4 g fat 2.6 g fiber 49.8 Cal

CHOCOLATE ICE CREAM

Ingredients

- 2 cups heavy cream

- 4 large egg yolks

- 10 sachets of calorie-free sweeteners

- ¼ cup cocoa powder (sugar-free)

- 2 unsweetened chocolate syrup Tbsp

- 1 tsp vanilla extract

Instructions

1. Heat the cream in a heavy saucepan over low heat. Beat the egg yolks 1 by 1. Cook over low heat, continually stirring until mixture covers the back of a spoon. Don't cook.

2. Keep away from heat. Add the sugar substitute, cocoa powder, chocolate syrup, and vanilla extract.

3. Cool to room temperature. Freeze.

Prep time: 20 min **Servings:** 4

Macros: 4.2 g net Carbs 3.2 g protein 24.6 g fat 1 g fiber 247.2 Cal

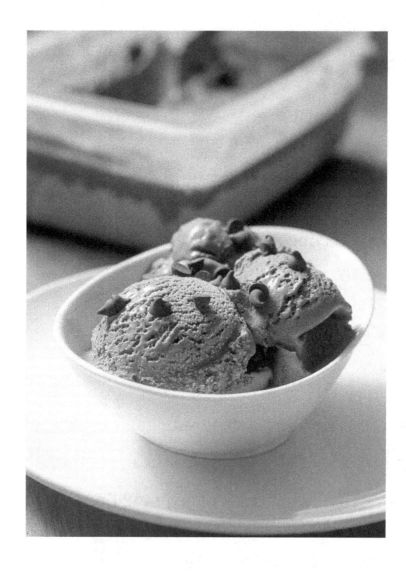

HAYSTACK WITH PEANUT BUTTER AND CHOCOLATE

Ingredients

- ¼ cup heavy cream

- 2 Tbsp unsalted butter bar

- 3 Tbsp cocoa powder (sugar-free)

- 2 Tbsp xylitol

- 1/16 pinch of Stevia

- 1/16 tsp salt

- ¼ cup natural creamy peanut butter

- 2/3 cup coconut, grated, sugar-free

Instructions

1. Combine cream, melted butter, cocoa powder, crystal sugar substitutes, and salt in a saucepan over medium heat. Bring to a boil then remove from heat. Add peanut butter and stir until it is absorbed.

2. Roast the coconut flakes in a saucepan at 350° For 5 min. Once it is roasted, add the chocolate mixture until it is covered.

3. Place Tbsp on waxed paper or a silicone mat on a tray to form 18 mounds. Let cool and harden or put in the fridge to dry quickly.

Prep time: 10 min **Servings:** 4

Macros: 1.1 g net Carbs 1.2 g protein 6.7 g fat 0.9 g fiber 74.9 Cal

PECAN AND CHOCOLATE CAKE

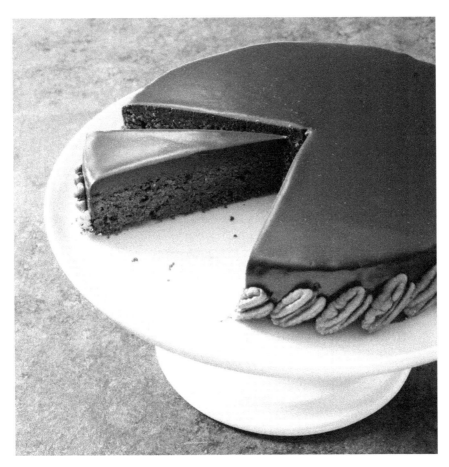

Ingredients

- 29 g of protein powdered milk chocolate

- 1 Tbsp coconut flour

- A pinch of salt

- 2 Tbsp canned pumpkin

- 1 Tbsp maple syrup (sugar-free)

- 1 Tbsp coconut oil

- 1 tsp vanilla extract

- ¼ cup chopped nuts

- 6 Tbsp Lily's Sugar-Free Chocolate Chips

- 1 tsp coconut oil

Instructions

1. In a small bowl, beat the protein powder, coconut flour, and salt.

2. Add the pumpkin puree, pancake syrup, coconut oil, and vanilla. Mix with a fork until it begins to crumble, then mix the finely chopped nuts.

3. Divide it into 9 balls, it's easier to do by wrapping it in a Tbsp. If the mixture crumbles too much and doesn't stick, add more pumpkin and a tsp at a time. Roll into solid balls and place them in an airtight container in the freezer for 30 min

4. Heat the chocolate and coconut oil at 30-second intervals until it melts in a microwave-safe glass container (or heat it

very carefully in a small box that fits into another container filled with ½ inch of water). Stir until completely melted. Place a piece of parchment paper on a drawer, set aside.

5. Remove the balls from the freezer and immerse the nuts with 2 forks in the chocolate and place them in the pan. If they are all covered, put them in the refrigerator for 30 min to cure them. After hardening, keep the balls for up to a week in an airtight container in the fridge.

Prep time: 25 min; **Servings:** 9

Macros: 1.8 g net Carbs 2.6 g protein 7.1 g fat 3.4 g fiber 82.8 Cal

CHOCOLATE NUT BUTTER COOKIE

Ingredients

- 16 Tbsp unsalted butter bar

- ½ cup sucralose sweetener (sugar substitute)

- 1 large egg (whole)

- 1 tsp vanilla extract

- 1 cup whole flour

- 3 tsp baking powder

- 2 cocoa powder Tbsp (sugar-free)

- ½ cup chopped pecans

Instructions

1. Preheat the oven to 325° F.

2. Beat butter and sugar substitute (½ cup) on medium speed with an electric mixer until smooth and fluffy, about 4 min.

3. Reduce the rate and add the egg, vanilla extract, and 1 tsp chocolate extract (optional). Scrape the bowl and add the soy flour, baking powder, cocoa powder, and nuts until everything is mixed.

4. Place the dough filling on ungreased baking sheets. Bake for 12 to 14 min, until the cookies are ready. Leave to cool on the leaves for 1 minute before transferring them to the racks to cool them completely.

Prep time: 20 min; **Servings:** 8

Macros: 1 g net Carbs 1.3 g protein 6 g fat 0.5 g fiber 62.9 Cal

CHOCOLATE AND MINT CUPCAKE

Ingredients

- 3 large eggs (whole)

- ¼ cup unsweetened coconut milk

- ¼ cup xylitol

- 1 tsp vanilla extract

- 3/4 tsp mint extract

- 7 Tbsp unsalted butter bar

- 4 Tbsp high-fiber organic coconut flour

- 2 cocoa powder Tbsp (sugar-free)

- ¼ tsp baking powder

- ¼ tsp salt

- 4 g of cream cheese

- 2 erythritol Tbsp

- 4 pieces Starlight Mint, sugar-free

Instructions

1. Sprinkle erythritol before preparing the frosting for this . Put 2 Tbsp in a blender and press 3-4 times to reduce to powder. To crush the mints, put them in a zipper bag, and hit them with a hammer.

2. Preheat the oven to 375° F. Prepare a muffin pan with 6 paper molds. Put aside.

3. Beat eggs in a medium bowl with coconut milk, granulated sugar substitute (xylitol), vanilla, mint extract, and 3 Tbsp melted butter. Put aside.

4. Combine coconut flour, cocoa powder, baking powder, and salt in a small bowl. Add to the beating egg mixture to incorporate all the ingredients for about a minute. Pour into the 6 paper cups, place in the oven and bake until they are entirely in the middle; about 15-18 min Place on a wire rack to cool.

5. Prepare the frosting: In a small bowl, beat the cream cheese with an electric mixer until smooth. Add ¼ cup (or 4 Tbsp)

of soft butter and continue beating for 1 minute. Add the erythritol powder; Beat for another minute, then add the mint extract and color as desired (optional; red is beautiful as in the photo and green is festive with red and white candies). Adjust the sweetness by adding a pinch of stevia if desired. Sprinkle with crushed mint candies.

Prep time:15 min; **Servings:** 4

Macros: 2.3 g net Carbs 5.7 g protein 23.6 g fat 2.3 g fiber 277.2 Cal

CHOCOLATE SOUFFLÉ

Ingredients

- 3 ⅓ Tbsp unsalted butter

- 3 Tbsp whole-grain soy flour

- ½ cup heavy cream

- ½ cup tap water

- 4 large eggs (whole)

- 2 tsp vanilla extract

- 2 g of sugar-free chocolate squares

- 3 Tbsp sucralose sweetener (sugar substitute)

Instructions

1. Preheat the oven to 350° F. Grease a 1½ quart soufflé plate with 1 tsp butter.

2. Melt the remaining 3 Tbsp butter in a small saucepan over medium heat. Beat the soy flour and cook for 3 min, stirring

constantly. Mix the cream with ½ cup water. Slowly add the cream mixture to the butter and soy flour. Boil 2-3 min on high heat. Remove from heat and add chocolate until it melts.

3. Separate the eggs into yolks and egg whites. Beat the egg yolks and vanilla in a large bowl for 2 min, until the color is slightly lighter. Add the chocolate mixture to the yolks and beat until well blended. Add the rest of the chocolate mixture and beat again until well blended.

4. In another large bowl, beat the egg whites with an electric mixer on high heat until frothy, about 2 min Slowly add the sugar substitute and continue beating until stiff peaks form, about 3 min more.

5. Using a rubber spatula, carefully fold half of the egg whites into the chocolate mixture until they come together. Add the remaining goals and fold them down until they are combined.

6. Pour into a greased dish and bake for 25 to 30 minutes, until it is puffy and ready, but still a bit wobbly in the middle. Serve hot.

Prep time: 15 min; **Servings:** 4

Macros: 3.6 g net Carbs 7.2 g protein 22.5 g fat 1.7 g fiber 242.1 Cal

CHOCOLATE CHEESECAKE

Ingredients

- 3/4 cup coconut, grated, sugar-free

- ½ cup almond flour

- 3 Tbsp cocoa powder (sugar-free)

- ¼ cup erythritol

- ¼ tsp salt

- ¼ cup unsalted butter bar

- 16 g of cream cheese

- 2 tsp vanilla extract

- ¼ tsp salt

- 18 Servings: of liquid Stevia

- 1 pack of powdered gelatin (sugar-free)

- 4 g of water, tap

- 1 ¼ cups heavy cream

- ¼ cup Lily's Sugar-Free Chocolate Chips

Instructions

10. Process the coconut, almond flour, cocoa powder, erythritol, salt, and butter in a food processor until they crumble. Press an 8-inch springform to cover the bottom and at least 1 inch on the sides. Place in the freezer until ready to fill.

11. The jelly flowers sprinkle on ½ cup water. Let stand for 1 minute, place in the microwave, and heat gently for 30 seconds, stirring to completely melt the jelly (do not overheat!). Set aside to cool.

12. Beat the cream cheese with the vanilla, salt, and stevia. Continue mixing until it is uniform. Then mix the hot mixture of gelatin and water and 1 cup heavy cream. Make sure the combination is uniform and divide it evenly into 2 bowls.

13. Heat ¼ cup cream in the microwave for 1 minute or up to 2 until it starts to boil. This is also possible on the stove. Place the chocolate chips in a bowl and pour and let stand for 1 to

2 min, beating until completely melted. Add to 1 of the reserved dishes.

14. Pour the vanilla pie dough into the pan with the crust. Then for the swirling chocolate dough, starting in the middle and working on the vanilla dough.

15. Place the cheesecake in the refrigerator and let it sit for at least 3 hours. Get out of the springform and enjoy it. This freezes very well, in the unlikely event that you end up.

Prep time: 20 min **Servings:** 9

Macros: 4.5 g net Carbs 7.3 g protein 33.5 g fat 1.9 g fiber 343.6 Cal

CHOCOLATE TART AND WHIPPED CREAM TAHINI

Ingredients

- 3 cups toasted and dried salted almonds

- ½ cup unsalted butter bar

- 1 ½ cups heavy cream

- 2 cocoa powder Tbsp (sugar-free)

- 4 Tbsp sucralose-based sweetener (sugar substitute)

- 1 cup organic tahini

- 1/8 cup, sliced almonds

Instructions

1. Preheat the oven to 350° F. Use a 12-well pan (or use a muffin pan with paper molds).

2. Press the salted almonds in a food processor until the most massive pieces are the size of a pea. Add the butter and press until everything is mixed. Spread the mixture on the Target

pan with your fingers until the sides and bottom are evenly covered. Bake for 10 min and let cool completely.

3. Heat the cream in a small saucepan until bubbles begin to form on the outside edges of the pan; constantly stir. Add the tahini, cocoa powder, and 3 Tbsp granular sugar substitute; Continue mixing until well mixed. Remove from heat, transfer to a small bowl and refrigerate for 20 min

4. When cool, remove the filling and stir again to mix. Divide the mixture among the pies.

5. Beat the cream and 1 Tbsp crystalline sugar substitute on medium speed in the bowl of an electric mixer equipped with the whisk until soft peaks appear. Place it with a spoon in a bag of pipes with a starting point and climb into a bubble bath. Garnish with flaked almonds. Keep cold until ready to serve or for at least 1 hour before serving.

Prep time:20 min **Servings:** 6

Macros: 6.1 g net Carbs 12.1 g protein 48.3 g fat 6.5 g fiber 500 Cal

CHOCOLATE AND NUTS

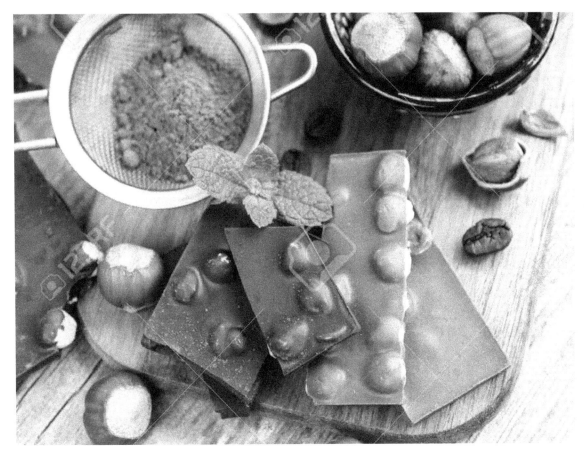

Ingredients

- 2 Tbsp 100% stone whole grain puff pastry

- 2 Tbsp whole-grain soy flour

- A pinch of baking powder

- 3/4 cup sucralose sweetener (sugar substitute)

- 1 ½ oz sugar-free cooking squares

- 5 Tbsp heavy cream

- 2 Tbsp unsalted butter bar

- 2 large eggs

- 1 tsp vanilla extract

- ¼ cup chopped English walnuts

Instructions

1. Preheat to 350° F. Roast the nuts lightly in an even layer on a baking sheet for 6 to 8 min. Chill, chop the nuts, and save.

2. Set the oven to 375° F. Cover 2 baking sheets with parchment paper or aluminum foil; put aside.

3. In a bowl, whisk 2 Tbsp whole wheat flour, 2 Tbsp soy flour, and baking powder; put aside.

4. In a large bowl of an electric mixer, beat eggs and sugar substitute over medium heat until soft and slightly thick.

5. Put the chocolate, cream, and butter in a microwave container; microwave over medium heat until butter melts

and the chocolate becomes soft (no need to melt completely), 1½ to 2 min Let sit for 5 min; Stir until smooth.

6. Gradually add the slightly hot chocolate mixture and vanilla extract to the egg mixture. Reduce speed to low and add flour mixture only until everything is combined. Cover and let cool 30 min

7. Place slightly rounded tsp, 1 inch apart, on the prepared sheet. Sprinkle the top of the cookies with nuts, lightly press the dough. Bake in the oven until cookies are ready but soft on top, 5½ to 6 min Cool the cookies on the baking sheet for 1 minute before moving them to the racks to cool them completely.

Prep time:20 min; **Servings:** 4

Macros: 0.9 g net Carbs 0.9 g protein 3.2 g fat 0.3 g fiber 35.7 Cal.

CHOCOLATE AND NUT BARS

Ingredients

- 3/4 cup sucralose sweetener (sugar substitute)

- ¼ cup chopped English walnuts

- 2 whole-grain soy flour Tbsp

- 3 large Protein

- 4 Tbsp unsalted butter bar

- 1 Tbsp cocoa powder (sugar-free)

- 2 tsp vanilla extract

Instructions

1. Preheat the oven to 400° F. Cover a baking sheet with a Silpat mat (available at most bakeries).

2. In a food processor, press the sugar substitute, nuts, and soy flour until they are finely ground, about 45 seconds. Put aside.

3. In a small bowl, combine egg whites, melted butter, cocoa powder, and extract until smooth. Pour the egg mixture into the dry ingredients and press for 15 to 20 seconds, scraping the bowl if necessary.

4. Place cookie dough by tsp on a baking sheet. Spread each cookie with the back of a spoon to a diameter of 2½ (it must be fragile). Bake for 7 to 8 min, until cooked through. Repeat this to make 30 cookies.

5. Remove the cookies from the baking sheet with a displaced spatula and bake on a rack; Repeat this with the remaining dough.

Prep time: 10 min; **Servings:** 8-10

Macros: 0.8 g net Carbs 0.7 g protein 2.3 g fat 0.2 g fiber 26.9 Cal

CHOCOLATE YOLES

Ingredients

- 1 ⅓ cup sucralose sweetener (sugar substitute)

- 5 Tbsp cocoa powder (sugar-free)

- 9 large eggs

- 2 Tbsp whole-grain soy flour

- ¼ tsp salt

- 1 ⅓ cup heavy cream

- 2 g of sugar-free chocolate squares

- 8 Tbsp unsalted butter bar

- ¼ tsp vanilla extract

Instructions

1. Preheat the oven to 375° F. Spray a pan with an oil spray; Covered with parchment, leaving a 2-inch border, spray again. Put aside.

2. In a large bowl, combine 1 cup sugar substitute, 4 Tbsp cocoa powder, and soy flour.

3. Beat the egg yolks in another large bowl with a fast electric mixer until you get a pale, fluffy yellow color, about 3 min Reduce speed to low and slowly mix the cocoa mixture until it is combined.

4. In another bowl, beat the egg whites and salt with an electric mixer on high speed until stiff peaks form, about 3 min.

5. Fold ⅓ of the Protein in the yolk mixture until they meet. Fold the remaining Protein. Roll out the dough evenly in a prepared pan. Bake for 15 min until the cake comes out when lightly touched and separated from the sides of the pan. Let the cake cool in a pan on a wire rack for 30 min to 1 hour.

6. While the cake cools, prepare the filling and frosting. For the filling, beat 1 cup cream and 1 ½ Tbsp sugar substitute in a medium bowl to form firm peaks (not to exceed).

7. For the icing, gradually mix ⅓ cup cream and melted chocolate in a large bowl. Beat the butter with an electric mixer on medium speed, 5 Tbsp sugar substitute, 1 Tbsp

cocoa powder, and vanilla. Beat until soft and fluffy, about 4 min Leave to cool in the refrigerator until needed.

8. When the cake is cold, slide it out of the pan with parchment underneath. Place on the counter. Spread the filling on the cake, with a ½ inch border. Roll the cake from the narrow end and use parchment. Cut 1-inch diagonal pieces at each end. Transfer the roll to a serving dish; Place the diagonal cut pieces on each side to form stem stumps. Put aside.

9. To assemble: use a small amount of glaze to fix the stumps to the main register. Freeze the entire log and insert the forks through the enamel to create a bark structure.

Prep time: 20 min; **Servings:** 18

Macros: 5.7 g net Carbs 8.2 g protein 28.9 g fat 1.8 g fiber 307.9 Cal

MINI CHOCOLATE AND CAPPUCCINO CUPCAKES

Ingredients

- 1 cup sliced almonds

- 1 cup whole flour

- 1 tsp baking powder

- ½ cup unsalted butter bar

- ½ cup sucralose sweetener (sugar substitute)

- 1 Tbsp cocoa powder (sugar-free)

- 1 tsp dry coffee (instant powder)

- 2 g or Tbsp chocolate whey protein

- 3 large eggs

Instructions

1. Preheat, the oven to 350° F. Spray mini muffin cups with cooking spray.

2. Process almonds in a food processor until they are finely ground. Add soy flour and baking powder; Impulse to combine.

3. In a large bowl, beat the butter and sugar substitute with an electric mixer until light, about 2 min Beat cocoa powder, coffee powder, and 2 oz Made from protein powder. Add the eggs 1 by 1. Mix the almond mixture with a spatula.

4. Bake for 20 min, until done.

Prep time: 15 min; **Servings:** 6

Macros: 7.2 g protein 9.9 g fat 1.4 g fiber 129 Cal 2.5 g net Carbs

431. CHOCOLATE AND COCONUT HAYSTACK

Ingredients

- 2 large Protein

- 1 cup sucralose sweetener (sugar substitute)

- 2 cocoa powder Tbsp (sugar-free)

- 2 cups unsweetened coconut flakes

- 2 Tbsp Hershey Unsweetened Chocolate Syrup

Instructions

1. Heat the oven to 325° F. Cover the baking sheets with aluminum foil.

2. Beat Protein to form weak to medium peaks; gradually add the sugar substitute and cocoa powder; Keep beating until firm peaks form. Stir in coconut and syrup.

3. Place the mixture with rounded tsp on the prepared baking sheets. Form small pyramids at the tips of wet fingers.

4. Bake for 12 min. Leave to cool for 1 minute before transferring them to the racks to cool them completely.

Prep time:15 min; **Servings:** 8

Macros: 1.4 g net Carbs 0.5 g protein 2.6 g fat 0.6 g fiber 29.8 Cal

CHOCOLATE AND GINGER CAKE

Ingredients

- 3/4 cup, half walnuts

- Bake 4 g of sugar-free chocolate squares

- ⅓ cup water

- ⅓ cup canola vegetable oil

- ¼ cup cocoa powder (sugar-free)

- ¼ cup whole wheat flour

- 2 ¼ cups sucralose sweetener (sugar substitute)

- 12 large eggs (whole)

- 2 tsp ginger (ground)

- ¼ tsp tartar

Instructions

6. Preheat to 350° F. Roast the nuts in an even layer on a baking sheet for 8 min. Leave to cool, cut the walnuts into thick pieces, and set aside.

7. Lower the oven to 325° F. Grease the bottom of a 10-inch tube and cover with parchment or waxed paper.

8. Put the chocolate and water in a microwave container; Cook in the microwave at high temperature for 1 to 2 min, until the chocolate melts, 1 minute apart. Stir until smooth, cold to hot and add oil; put aside.

9. Squeeze the nuts, cocoa powder, and soy flour in a food processor until nuts are finely ground. Beat the egg yolks in a large bowl with a sugar substitute at high speed with an electric mixer until they are soft and fluffy, about 5 min Add the melted chocolate, nut mixture and ginger.

10. In another large bowl, beat the egg whites and tartar on medium speed with an electric mixer until fluffy. Gradually add the remaining sugar substitute, beating until stiff peaks form. Use a rubber spatula to fold a third of the meringue into the egg yolk mixture to become lighter; fold the rest of the meringue until it is combined.

11. Pour batter evenly into prepared pan and bake until a toothpick in the center of the cake comes out clean, about 45 min Let the cake cool for 30 min before removing it from the pan.

12. Removal: Place a knife along the inside and outside edges of the cake, place a wire rack or plate on the pan and turn. Remove the mold and remove the paper. Let cool completely before cutting.

Prep time: 20 min **Servings:** 16

Macros: 5.3 g Net Carbs 7.1 g Protein 15.9 g Fat 2.1 g Fiber 187.5 Cal

CHOCOLATE MINT MOUSSE CAKE

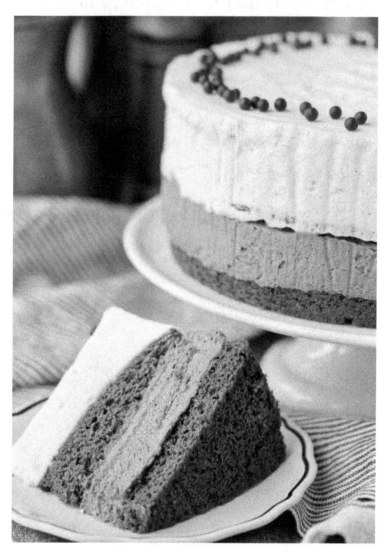

Ingredients

4. 1 cup heavy cream

5. 2 tsp vanilla extract

6. ½ oz coffee (instant powder)

7. 1 ¼ cups whole wheat flour

8. ½ cup cocoa powder (sugar-free)

9. ½ cup, half walnuts

10. ½ tsp baking powder

11. ½ tsp salt

12. 1 cup unsalted butter bar

13. 1 cup sucralose sweetener (sugar substitute)

14. 4 large eggs (whole)

Instructions

6. Preheat the oven to 325° F. Grease 2 8-inch round cake pans with spray oil.

7. Combine cream, vanilla, and coffee in a small bowl. Put aside. Combine soy flour, cocoa, chopped nuts, baking powder, and salt in a medium bowl. Put aside. In a large bowl, with an electric mixer on medium speed, beat the butter with half the sugar substitute until soft and fluffy, about 5 min

8. Separate the eggs into yolks and egg whites. Add egg yolks 1 by 1, beat well and scrape the sides of the bowl after each addition. Add the thick cream mixture and beat until well blended. Reduce the speed of the blender on low speed and slowly add the dry ingredients, a third at a time, beating until they are combined. Put aside.

9. Beat the egg whites in another large bowl until soft tips appear, about 3 min Add the remaining sugar substitute and beat until stiff peaks form, about 1 minute longer. Fold the egg whites in a chocolate dough with a rubber spatula and mix well after each addition.

10. Divide the dough into prepared shapes; Smooth top. Bake for 20 min, or until the cake comes out when you touch it in the middle. Let cool in saucepans on racks for 5 min; invest in frames to cool completely, about 2 hours.

11. To assemble the cake: Cut the rounded top of each cupcake. Place a layer of cake on a serving platter, slicing it down. Spread the top with half the foam and leave a half-edge. Place the cut side of the other layer of cake on the mousse and press gently be careful not to let out the foam. Cover it with

the remaining foam and turn decorative. Garnish with raspberries and mint leaves.

Prep time:30 min; **Servings:** 8

Macros: 11.4 g of net Carbs 25.8 g of protein 67.9 g oFat 4.3 g oFiber 754.5 Cal.

CHOCOLATE AND PEANUT

Ingredients

- 1 Tbsp cocoa powder (sugar-free)

- 1 Tbsp ⅓ natural creamy peanut butter less sodium and sugar

- 2 tsp sucralose sweetener (sugar substitute)

- 2 Tbsp heavy cream

Instructions

1. Mix 1 Tbsp unsweetened cocoa powder, 1 Tbsp soft peanut butter and 1 sachet of sweetener with a spatula.

2. Beat 2 Tbsp heavy cream until soft peaks form.

3. Gently add the peanut butter mixture.

Prep time:5 min; **Servings:** 1

Macros: 4.9 g net Carbs 5.2 g protein 20.3 g fat 2.8 g fiber 223.5 Cal

CHOCOLATE AND RUM CAKE

Ingredients

- 3/4 cup soy flour

- 2 cocoa powder Tbsp

- 1 tsp baking powder

- 4 Tbsp unsalted butter bar

- 3 g of cream cheese

- 1 Tbsp sour cream (cultivated)

- 1 ½ cups heavy cream

- 2 oz water

- 3 oz squares of baking chocolate without sugar

- ¼ cup cocoa powder (sugar-free)

- 2 large egg yolks

- 3/4 cup sucralose sweetener (sugar substitute)

- 1 tsp rum extract

- 1 tsp vanilla extract

- 3 tsp sucralose (Splenda)

Instructions

1. For the cake batter: mix the soy flour, 2 Tbsp cocoa powder, baking powder, butter, 3 oz cream cheese, and sour cream in a food processor; only turn into a mixed dough and held together. Form a ball then form a disc. Wrap it well in plastic and let it cool for 20 min

2. Save a quarter of the dough. Squeeze small dough balls (½ inch) from the rest of the mixture and spread them evenly over the bottom and sides of a 9-inch cake pan. Press mixture evenly on the bottom and sides with your fingers to form a crust. With a reserved mixture and using the same method, build a border around the upper edge of the crust; Press lightly on the edge of the dough with the teeth of a fork to create a winning side. Pierce the bottom with a fork. Leave to cool in the freezer for 30 min

3. Heat the oven to 425° F. Press gently on the edge of the crust with small strips of aluminum foil (too brown). Store without pressing aluminum foil over the entire coat. Bake for 10 min Lower the oven temperature to 375° F and bake for 10 min Carefully remove the carp and the rough skin from the edge of the bark (the side will be very fragile). Return to oven and bake until golden brown for about 1 minute. Let cool entirely on a wire rack.

4. For the garnish: place 3/4 cup cream, 2 Tbsp water, chocolate, and cocoa powder in a medium saucepan. Cook over medium heat, beating, until the chocolate melts and the mixture is smooth, 5 to 7 min Away from heat; set aside.

5. In a medium bowl, whisk together the egg yolks, ¼ cup cream, the remaining 2 Tbsp water, and the sugar substitute until well blended. Beat the chocolate mixture well. Gradually mix a third of the chocolate mixture into the egg yolk mixture; Add to the pan with the rest of the chocolate mixture and mix to combine. Reheat and cook over medium heat, continually stirring for 3 min Remove from heat and allow to cool to room temperature. Add rum and vanilla extracts.

6. In a medium bowl, with an electric mixer in the middle, beat the remaining ½ cup cream until soft peaks form. Fold the chocolate mixture, fold only until it mixes, and no streaks appear. Pour into prepared cake batter and smooth the top. Let cool until ready, at least 4 hours. (The cake can be prepared at this point and cooled overnight.) Cover with whipped cream and decorate with mint leaves (optional).

Prep time:30 min; **Servings:** 16

Macros: 4.2 g net Carbs 3.8 g protein 17.4 g fat 1.8 g fiber 181.9 Cal

CHOCOLATE AND SOUR CREAM CUPCAKES

Ingredients

- 1 ⅓ cups whole grain soy flour

- 1 ¼ cups sucralose sweetener (sugar substitute)

- ⅓ cup cocoa powder (sugar-free)

- 1 tsp baking powder

- ¼ tsp salt

- 6 large eggs (whole)

- 8 g of sour cream

- 2 Tbsp vegetable oil

- ¼ cup tap water

- 2 tsp vanilla extract

Instructions

3. Preheat the oven to 350° F. Grease a 12-cup muffin pan with spray oil.

4. Combine soy flour, sugar substitute, cocoa powder, baking powder, and salt in a large bowl. Mix to combine.

5. Combine eggs, sour cream, water, oil, and vanilla in another large bowl. Add wet ingredients to dry ingredients, mix with a wooden spoon until they are combined.

6. Divide the batter into a greased muffin pan and bake for 15 to 20 min, until the stick in the middle of a cake comes out clean. Let the fresh cupcakes in the pan for 5 min Loosen the muffins and remove them with a thin metal spatula and place them on a wire rack to cool them completely.

Prep time: 15 min **Servings:** 12

Macros: 6.2 g Net Carbs 8.6 g Protein 11.7 g Fat 2.1 g Fiber 166.5 Cal

MACADAMIA NUT CHOCOLATE ICE CREAM SANDWICH

Ingredients

- ½ cup salted butter

- 3/4 cup sucralose sweetener

- 2 tsp vanilla extract

- 3 large eggs (whole)

- 1 cup flour mixture (cups)

- ½ tsp baking powder

- 5 Tbsp Lily's sugar-free chocolate chips

- 3 cups heavy cream

- 3 large egg yolks

- ¼ tsp salt

- ½ cup whole or half macadamia nuts

- ½ tsp pure almond extract

Instructions

4. Preheat the oven to 375° F.

5. For cookies: you need 1 cup of the flour mixture. Mix soft butter, ½ cup crystalline sugar substitute, and 1 tsp vanilla until smooth. Add an egg and continue mixing until it is thick and creamy. Add the flour mixture and baking powder mixture to a smooth batter. Fold the chocolate chips. Wear the dough to make 20 balls of the same size. Place 2 inches apart in a pan lined with parchment paper, lightly flat and bake for 10-12 min until light brown. Set aside to cool.

6. For the macadamia nut ice cream: for the heavy cream into a 3-liter thick bottom pan and place over medium heat. Bring to a boil, stirring regularly so that the cream does not boil. Keep away from heat.

7. Place 2 eggs, 3 egg yolks, ¼ cup sugar and salt substitute in a large bowl. Beat with a hand blender or blender until it is thick and smooth.

8. Remove a cup of hot cream from the pan with a ladle and gradually mix in the egg mixture (this will temper the eggs,

so they don't curdle). Beat for the hot egg mixture into the remaining cream in a saucepan.

9. Place over medium heat and beat until slightly thicker, 1 to 2 min For into a clean bowl, mix 1 tsp vanilla and almond extract; Let stand until the cream is completely cooled to room temperature, about 1 ½ hours. Let cool for 2 hours, until it is cold, or cover with plastic wrap and overnight in the refrigerator.

10. Freeze in the ice-cream maker according to the manufacturer's instructions. Add the chopped macadamia nuts 15 min before the end of the freezing process.

11. To make sandwiches: place 10 cookies, face down, on the work surface. Use a scoop of ice cream, work fast, place ¼ cup ice cream on each cookie. Cover each with a different cookie, bottom down.

12. Wrap each sandwich tightly in plastic wrap and place it in the freezer. Freeze for at least 4 hours (ice is soft) or overnight (for firmer sandwiches). It can be stored in the fridge for up to 1 month.

Prep time:30 min **Servings:** 10

Macros: 6.8 g of net Carbs 11 g of protein 47.1 g oFat 5 g oFiber 490.9 of Cal

CHOCOLATE DONUT DELIGHT

Ingredients

- 1 large egg (whole)

- 4 g of almond butter

- 2 cocoa powder Tbsp (sugar-free)

- 6 tsp erythritol

- ¼ tsp baking powder

- ¼ tsp baking powder

- ¼ tsp salt

- ½ can (14 oz) coconut cream

- 2 tsp vanilla extract

Instructions

1. Preheat the oven to 350° F. Prepare a 6-well donut platter with a non-stick spray.

2. Put all the ingredients in a blender or food processor, press several times, and scrape the bowl between the legumes.

3. Pour into a donut tray and bake for 13 min Leave to cool in the pan for 10 min, then light a rack to cool completely.

Prep time:5 min; **Servings:** 3

Macros: 9.1 g of net Carbs 5 g of protein 19.1 g oFat 1.3 g oFiber 205.5 of Cal

CHOCOLATE FONDUE

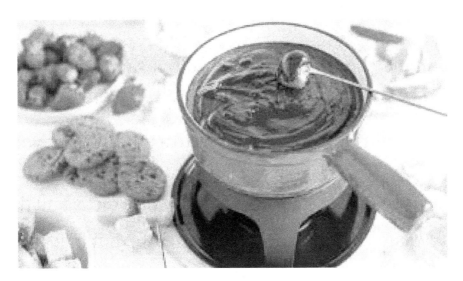

Ingredients

- 3 fresh kiwis

- 18 medium-sized strawberries (1-1 / 4 "in diameter), fresh

- 16 Tbsp Lily's sugar-free chocolate chips

- 2/3 cup heavy cream

- ½ fluid oz (without ice) cognac

Instructions

1. Make the low-carb cake of your choice. The following s work well for this : chocolate and ginger cake, spicy snack cake, or the cupcake portion with strawberries and cream. Cut the

low-carb cake into 1-inch pieces, leave the strawberries whole and peel the kiwis and cut them into 12-15 pieces.

2. Combine chocolate and cream in a saucepan and cook over medium heat, stirring until chocolate is melted. Add the cognac and pour the mixture into a fondue pan over low heat.

3. Discard the fruit and cake with fondue forks and dip them in chocolate. If the chocolate begins to bubble, it is too hot; lower the heat or extinguish the flames for a few minutes.

Prep time: 25 min; **Servings:** 20

Macros: 9.1 g net Carbs 2.9 g protein 16.6 g fat 15.4 g fiber 196.7 Cal

CINNAMON CHURRITO

Ingredients

- ½ cup blanched almond flour

- 2 Tbsp high-fiber organic coconut flour

- ¼ tsp baking powder (straight phosphate, double effect)

- 2 tsp cinnamon

- A pinch of salt

- ½ cup unsweetened coconut milk

- 1 Tbsp unsalted butter

- 3 Tbsp xylitol

- 1 large egg (whole)

Instructions

1. Prepare a large skillet or fryer with 2-3 inches of oil. Heat to 350° F. In a small bowl, combine the almond flour, coconut

flour, baking powder, 1 tsp cinnamon, and salt. Mix well and set aside.

2. Boil the coconut milk, butter, and 1 Tbsp xylitol in a small saucepan. Remove from heat and add the flour mixture, stirring until it is very thick and forms a ball. Let cool 5 min

3. Once it is cold, add 1 egg and mix in a very thick dough, about 1 minute. Place 4 to 8 Tbsp at a time in the fryer and fry on the outside until golden and crisp; about 3-4 min; turn halfway. Repeat this until all the dough has been used. It makes about 16 balls. Put them on a paper towel as soon as they are finished.

4. Press the remaining 2 Tbsp xylitol with 1 tsp cinnamon 1-2 times in a blender until the grains of xylitol are slightly smaller. When you are done with each batch, roll the xylitol and cinnamon mixture until it is evenly covered and place it in a bowl. Take advantage immediately, or they can be stored at room temperature for 1 day. It can also be frozen for 3 months or chilled for up to 1 week. 2 scoops per serving

Prep time: 10 min; **Servings:** 8

Macros: 1.4 g of net Carbs 2.6 g of protein 6.1 g oFat 1.8 g oFiber 85.1 Cal Cal

CINNAMON CUSTARD

Ingredients

- 2 cups heavy cream

- ½ cinnamon tsp

- 2 large eggs (whole)

- 2 large egg yolks

- ½ cup sucralose sweetener (sugar substitute)

- A pinch of salt

- ½ tsp vanilla extract

- 18 tsp unsweetened flavored syrup, caramel

Instructions

3. Prepare the day before, cover with plastic wrap, and cool.

4. Combine cream and cinnamon in a heavy medium saucepan.

5. Heat over medium heat and continuously beat to mix the cinnamon with the cream until the cream begins to smoke.

6. Do not boil away from heat.

7. Heat the oven to 300° F.

8. Combine eggs, egg yolks, sugar substitute, and salt in a medium bowl until pale yellow and somewhat thick.

9. Beat the hot cream gradually. When all the cream has been added, add the vanilla extract.

10. Pour about ½ cup the cream mixture into each of the 6 cups of 4-oz custard (or for the whole mixture into a 2-quart round baking dish).

11. Place the cups or baking dish in a roasting pan.

12. Gently pour enough boiling water (about 4 cups) into the pan until half the cups or baking dish is halfway.

13. Cook until the cream is slightly loose in the middle, about 30 min (Cook the baking dish for another 5 min).

14. Carefully remove the cups from the double boiler with a kitchen glove.

15. Serve hot, at room temperature or cold, mix each serving with 1 Tbsp (3 tsp each) of caramel syrup.

Prep time: 20 min; **Servings:** 6

Macros: 4.4 g of net Carbs 4.6 g of protein 32.5 g oFat 0.1 g oFiber 324.6 of Cal

CINNAMON FAN CUPS

Ingredients

8. 2 large eggs

9. 1 cup heavy cream

10. 2/3 cup (8 fluid oz) of water, press

11. 3 Tbsp maple syrup (sugar-free)

12. ½ cinnamon tsp

Instructions

1. Preheat the oven to 325° F.

2. Beat the eggs in a large bowl.

3. Boil the cream, water, pancake syrup, and cinnamon in a small saucepan. Gradually mix the cream mixture in the eggs and return to the pan.

4. Pour the mixture through a sieve into 4 6-oz molds or custard cups. Place the cups in a large skillet; Carefully pour boiling water into the pan to reach half the cups.

5. Cover the entire pan with aluminum foil and bake for 35 min, until the cream is in the middle. Remove from the oven and let stand in the pan for 15 min

6. Remove the cups from the pan and put in the refrigerator for 2 hours, covered with a plastic sheet before serving.

Prep time: 20 min; **Servings:** 4

Macros: 2.1 g Carbs 4.4 g Protein 24.5 g Fat 0.2 g Fiber 245.6 Cal.

CINNAMON ALMOND MERINGUE

Ingredients

- ½ cup whole almonds

- 10 packages of sucralose sweetener (sugar substitute)

- 3 large Protein

- A pinch of of tartar

- ½ tsp pure almond extract

- ½ tsp cinnamon

Instructions

7. Preheat the oven to 200° F. Cover a baking sheet with aluminum foil.

8. Cut the nuts with a sugar substitute in a food processor until nuts are finely ground.

9. In a large bowl, with an electric mixer at high speed, beat the egg whites until soft tips form. Add cream of tartar, the

almond extract, and the cinnamon whisk until stiff peaks form. Carefully stir in the nut mixture.

10. Spoon 8 mounds evenly distributed on a prepared baking sheet. Make a floor in the middle of each with the back of the spoon.

11. Bake the meringues on the center rack of the oven for 1 hour 30 min, until they are golden and scorched. Turn off the oven and let the meringues dry in the oven until they cool. Remove the meringues from the aluminum foil.

Prep time: 20 min; **Servings:** 8

Macros: 2 g net Carbs 3.3 g protein 4.6 g fat 1.1 g fiber 64 Cal

CHOCOLATE CUPCAKES

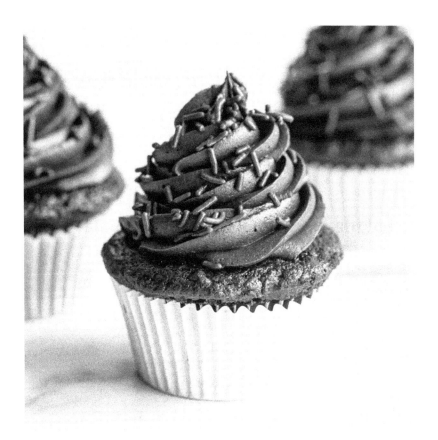

Ingredients

- 1 cup unsalted butter bar

- 9 Tbsp xylitol

- 3 large eggs (whole)

- 4 tsp vanilla extract

- 5 fluid oz cream

- 3 tap water Tbsp

- 2 Tbsp high-fiber organic coconut flour

- 1 cup blanched almond flour

- ⅓ cup cocoa powder (sugar-free)

- ½ tsp baking powder (straight phosphate, double effect)

- ¼ tsp baking powder

- ¼ tsp salt

- Bake 2 g of sugar-free chocolate squares

- 1 tsp dry coffee (instant powder)

Instructions

This is suitable for all phases except for the first 2 weeks of nut induction. Xylitol is generally in granular form and is the preferred sweetener for taste when using chocolate. Measure first, then spray the xylitol in a blender before using it in this

Cupcakes:

1. Preheat the oven to 325 ° F. Cover a muffin pan with 12 papers or aluminum foil.

2. Beat ½ cup soft butter with 5 Tbsp xylitol until pale and fluffy; about 3 min Add the eggs 1 at a time until they are completely absorbed, then add 3 tsp vanilla, 2 oz (about ¼ cup) of heavy cream, water, and flour of coconut. Mix well.

3. Combine almond flour, cocoa powder, baking powder, baking powder consistently, and salt in a separate bowl. Add to wet ingredients and beat until smooth and thick. Divide among muffin tins and bake for 20-25 min or until they are fully cooked, be careful not to overcook. Otherwise, they will become bitter. Leave to cool in the muffin pan for 5 min, then place on a wire rack to cool.

Cream:

4. Melt the chocolate with about 20 ml of heavy cream in the microwave at 20-second intervals. Stir and let cool completely. Once cool, mix 4 Tbsp xylitol. Put aside.

5. In a tiny bowl, stir in 1 tsp vanilla, 1 tsp cocoa powder (optional), and 1 tsp instant coffee. Put aside.

6. Transfer the fresh chocolate to a medium bowl and beat with the remaining ½ cup butter on medium speed until it becomes lighter. Add the reserved vanilla mixture and whisk to combine.

7. Place the frosting on the cupcakes using a pastry bag with a cut corner. Decorate with chocolate candy and peanuts if desired.

Prep time: 10 min; **Servings:** 6

Macros: 3.1 g net Carbs 5.3 g protein 28.7 g fat 2.9 g fiber 310.7 Cal

COCONUT COOKIES

Ingredients

- ¼ cup, whole hazelnuts

- ½ cup whole wheat flour

- ⅓ cup dried coconut

- 2 large Protein

- 1/8 can of Seltzer water

- 1 ½ tsp coconut extract

- ½ tsp vanilla extract

- ½ tsp salt

- 8 Tbsp unsalted butter bar

- 7 Tbsp sucralose sweetener (sugar substitute)

Instructions

4. Preheat the oven to 350° F. Roast the hazelnuts in an even layer on a baking sheet for 8 min Leave to cool, cut into large pieces, and set aside.

5. Increase the oven temperature to 375° F. Grease a baking sheet with an oil spray.

6. Mix in a large bowl of soy flour, unsweetened coconut, hazelnuts, egg whites, 2 Tbsp seltzer, 1 ½ tsp coconut and ½ tsp vanilla extract, salt, butter, and sugar substitute. Mix well.

7. Place 1 rounded spoon (12 cookies) on a prepared baking sheet. Bake for 20 min or until light brown. Let the cookies cool on the baking sheet for 1 minute before transferring them to the racks to cool them completely.

Prep time:8 min; **Servings:** 6

Macros: 2.1 g of net Carbs 3 g of protein 12.2 g oFat 1.2 g oFiber 130 of Cal

COCONUT LEMON ICE CREAM WITH BLACKBERRY AND PEACH COMPOTE

Ingredients

- 9 Servings: of coconut cream

- 1/16 tsp salt

- 4 large egg yolks

- ½ cup xylitol

- 1/16 pinch of Stevia

- 3 lemon zest tsp

- ½ cup lemon juice

- 4 portions of blackberries with peach and compote

Instructions

1. Use the to make a blackberry and peach compote. The suggests 4 Servings: of the compote, 1 serving is ¼ cup.

2. Combine 2 cups of coconut cream and a pinch of salt in a medium saucepan. Heat until boiling. While the coconut cream is heating, mix the egg yolks, granulated sugar substitutes, and lemon zest. Beat to combine.

3. Slowly for the coconut milk into the egg yolk mixture, beating continuously. Transfer the mixture to dip pan over medium heat. Cook, stirring continuously, until it reaches 170 ° F and starts covering the back of a wooden spoon, do not allow the mixture to boil.

4. Place the mixture on an ice water bath and add 1 cup remaining coconut cream and ½ cup lemon juice. Let cool to room temperature and transfer to the refrigerator. Store in the fridge overnight or for at least 4 hours to intensify and cool the flavors.

5. Once cool, place it in the refrigerator and follow the manufacturer's instructions for making ice cream. Take advantage of it immediately or put it in a freezer and freeze it for at least 4 hours or at most a month. Makes about 1 liter of ice cream, 1 serving equals about ½ cup. Before serving, place in the refrigerator for 20-30 min Dip the scoop of ice in

hot water and help the ice to serve. Cover with 2 Tbsp blackberry compote and peach.

Prep time: 45 min; **Servings:** 9

Macros: 5.2 g net Carbs 2.8 g protein 21.5 g fat 1.8 g fiber 256.5 Cal

COCONUT MACAROON

Ingredients

- 4 large Protein

- 2/3 cup sucralose sweetener (sugar substitute)

- ½ tsp vanilla extract

- ¼ tsp salt

- 2 cups coconut, grated, sugar-free

Instructions

1. Heat the oven to 325° F. Spray 2 baking sheets with a spray of oil.

2. Beat the Protein at medium speed with an electric mixer until medium peaks form. Gradually add the sugar substitute, vanilla extract, and salt. Speed up and continue beating until firm (but not dry) peaks form.

3. Use a rubber spatula, double coconut.

4. Form spoon-sized heaps on prepared baking sheets. Bake for 15 min.

5. Leave to cool for 1 minute on the leaves before carefully transferring them to the racks so that they cool completely.

Prep time: 20 min; **Servings:** 8

Macros: 1.2 g net Carbs 0.8 g protein 3.9 g fat 0.7 g fiber 46.9 Cal

COCONUT PANNA SKULLOTTA

Ingredients

- 1 can (14 oz) coconut cream

- 2 sachets of gelatin, sugar-free

- 2 cups heavy cream

- ½ cup sucralose sweetener (sugar substitute)

- 1 tsp vanilla extract

- 2 tsp coconut extract

Instructions

1. Pour 1 cup coconut milk or coconut cream into a medium bowl. Sprinkle with gelatin and let sit until tender, about 1 minute

2. Mix the rest of the coconut milk in a small saucepan with the heavy cream. Heat over medium heat, stirring until tiny bubbles begin to form along the sides of the pan. For over the

jelly mixture. Add the sucralose and mix well. Let cool to room temperature.

3. Once the mixture has cooled, add the vanilla and 2 tsp coconut extract. Spray a 4 cup form of aerosol oil, for the gelatin mixture, cover with plastic wrap and store overnight or until ready; Minimum 4 hours

4. To serve, separate the panna cotta from the pan around the edges and place it carefully on a plate. Garnish with unsweetened grated coconut if desired.

Prep time:25 min **Servings:** 8

Macros: 3.2 g of net Carbs 2.6 g of protein 21.5 g oFat 0 g oFiber 210.4 of Cal

COCONUT PIE

Ingredients

- 5 ½ g of almonds

- 1 3/4 cups coconut, grated, sugar-free

- 3/4 cup sucralose sweetener

- 1 large protein

- 1 can (14 oz) coconut cream

- ½ cup heavy cream

- 6 large eggs (whole)

- 1 large yolk egg

- ¼ tsp salt

- 1 tsp vanilla extract

- 1 tsp coconut extract

Instructions

1. For the crust: Heat the oven to 350° F. Grind the almonds in the flour. Combine almond flour, 1 cup grated coconut, ¼ cup sugar substitute, and egg whites. If the coconut mixture is too dry to keep it together, add 1 to 2 tsp water, a few drops at a time until the dough retains its shape when it collects.

2. Press the top and bottom of a cake pan to form a crust. Bake 15 min until lightly browned. Remove from the oven; put aside. Increase the oven temperature to 450° F.

3. For the garnish: blanch the milk and coconut cream in a medium saucepan; Cool slightly. In a large bowl, beat with an electric mixer at medium speed (or with a whisk), eggs, and egg yolk until fluffy. Beat ½ cup sugar substitute, salt, vanilla, and coconut extract. Slowly beat in the coconut milk mixture.

4. Add 3/4 cup grated coconut and stir gently. For the filling into prepared crust. Bake for 5 min at 450° F. Lower the temperature to 350° F and bake for another 15 min or until a knife near the center comes out clean. Leave to cool on a rack at room temperature, then transfer to the refrigerator to cool completely.

Prep time:30 min; **Servings:** 8

Macros: 8.5 g net Carbs 12.3 g protein 42.7 g fat 4.6 g fiber 475 Cal

COCONUT COOKIES WITH BERRIES AND CREAM

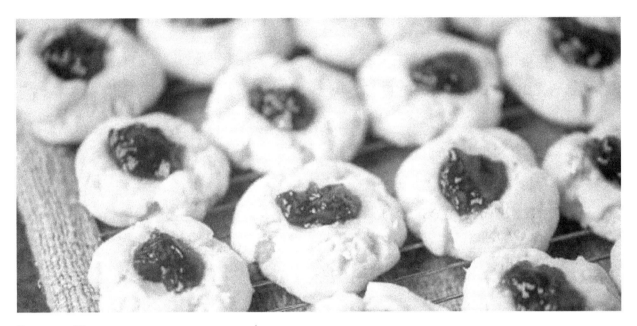

Ingredients

- ¼ cup whole wheat flour

- 1 tsp baking powder

- ⅓ cup coconut, grated, sugar-free

- 4 Tbsp sucralose-based sweetener

- 3 Tbsp unsalted butter bar

- 1 large egg (whole)

- 1 tsp coconut extract

- 1 2/3 cup heavy cream

- 1 tsp vanilla extract

- 1 ¼ cups red raspberries

- 1 ¼ cup strawberries

- ½ cup blueberries

Instructions

1. Heat oven to 375° F. In a large bowl, combine soy flour, baking powder, ¼ cup coconut, 3 Tbsp sugar substitute, and melted butter. Make a well in the center and add the egg, coconut extract and 2/3 cup heavy cream. Beat the liquid ingredients until they are mixed, then combine with the dry mixture and mix only until they are mixed.

2. Place the mixture on a baking sheet with a quarter cup slightly rounded to make 6 heaps. Form with your fingertips each in 2½ turns; Divide and sprinkle the rest of the coconut on top. Cover with plastic wrap and leave in the refrigerator for 20 min Bake for 12 min, or until edges are lightly golden and firm to the touch. Put in a rack and let cool completely.

3. Meanwhile, beat with an electric mixer on medium heat 1 cup remaining thick cream, 1 Tbsp sugar substitute, and vanilla extract in soft peaks. Beat 1 Tbsp unsweetened jam (if used) in a medium bowl until smooth; add raspberries, sliced strawberries, and blueberries and stir gently until covered.

4. Divide the cakes in half horizontally to serve. Spread ⅓ cup whipped cream on the bottom of each cupcake. Place ½ cup berries on the whipped cream and cover with the top of the cake. Cover with a Tbsp whipped cream, if desired.

Prep time: 20 min; **Servings:** 4

Macros: 9.2 g net Carbs 5 g protein 35.7 g fat 3.7 g fiber 383.3 Cal.

COCONUT FINGERPRINT

Ingredients

- 2/3 cup Brazil nuts

- ½ cup coconut, grated, sugar-free

- ½ cup whole wheat flour

- 2 ½ Tbsp sucralose-based sweetener

- ½ cup unsalted butter bar

- 1 large egg (whole)

- 1 large egg yolk

- 1 tsp coconut extract

- 3 Tbsp blackberries

Instructions

1. Preheat the oven to 375° F.

2. Squeeze ½ cup coconut and walnuts in a food processor until finely ground, about 1 minute. Add soy flour and sugar substitute and press to combine.

3. Add the butter and squeeze until mixture looks like a full meal, about 30 seconds longer. Add the egg, yolk and extract and press until the dough comes together for about 1 minute.

4. Scrape the dough in a bowl, cover, and let cool for at least 3 hours until it is firm. Roll the dough into 36 balls and place them on an ungreased baking sheet. Dip your thumb in lukewarm water and make an impression in the middle of each shot, forming a donut shape (but not pressing ultimately).

5. Fill each level with a quarter of a tsp jam. Cook until golden brown, about 6 min Let cool on baking sheet for 1 minute before placing on a wire rack to cool completely.

Prep time:20 min; **Servings:** 4

Macros: 0.9 g net Carbs 1.3 g protein 5.7 g fat 0.7 g fiber 60 Cal

CHOCOLATE AND COCONUT TRUFFLE

Ingredients

- 3/4 cup heavy cream

- 2 Tbsp sucralose sweetener (sugar substitute)

- 2 Tbsp unsalted butter bar

- 14 g of unsweetened chocolate chips

- 3 oz squares of baking chocolate without sugar

- 3/4 tsp vanilla extract

- 1 cup coconut, grated, sugar-free

- 4 Tbsp cashews, whole, raw

Instructions

1. Combine cream, sugar substitute and butter in a small saucepan. Bring to a boil. Place the chopped chocolate in a medium bowl; For the hot cream mixture over the chocolate. Let sit for 5 min

2. Gently stir the chocolate mixture until the chocolate completely melts. Add extract and ½ cup coconut. Let cool until firm, about 1 hour and 45 min, occasionally stirring (the truffles will be more natural to shape if the mixture is not too firm).

3. Grill the remaining ½ cup coconut in a dry skillet over medium heat, frequently stirring, until lightly browned; Put in a bowl and let cool.

4. Roll the chocolate mixture into 32 balls the size of large balls. Roll half the balls in the cashews and the other half in toasted coconut. Place in layers of waxed paper in an airtight container. You can keep in the refrigerator for up to a week.

Prep time:30 min; **Servings:** 16

Macros: 2.3 g of net Carbs 1.9 g of protein 10.6 g oFat 1.6 g oFiber 130.4 of Cal

COCONUT LIME MOUSSE

Ingredients

- 2 g cream cheese

- 4 packages of sucralose sweetener

- ¼ cup fresh lime juice

- 1 tsp coconut extract (sugar-free)

- 1 cup heavy cream

Instructions

1. With an electric mixer, mix 2 oz soft cream cheese and 4 packets of granulated sugar substitute (equivalent to 8 tsp) to a smooth mass.

2. Slowly add ¼ cup lime juice and beat until creamy.

3. Beat 1 tsp coconut extract (you can use vanilla if coconut is not available) and 1 cup heavy cream until fluffy.

4. Place in 4 bowls, sprinkle with 1 Tbsp unsweetened coconut flakes (optional, don't forget to add. 4 g of NC Carbs), and keep until ready to serve.

Prep time:10 min; **Servings:** 4

Macros: 4.3 g net Carbs 2.4 g protein 27 g fat 0.1 g fiber 261.9 Cal

COEUR A LA CREME

Ingredients

- 4 g of cream cheese

- ¼ cup cottage cheese

- ¼ cup sour cream

- ½ cup heavy cream

- 4 tsp sucralose sweetener

- 1 tsp vanilla extract

- A pinch of salt

Instructions

1. Prepare the molds: make several holes in the bottom of the disposable muffin cups. Wet the mesh, drain it, and fold it in half. Place a mesh on the box and press it into shapes, leaving a 2-inch border along the edge of the box. Put aside.

2. To prepare a heart: press the cream cheese, cottage cheese, and sour cream in a food processor until smooth and scrape the sides if necessary. Transfer to a large bowl and set aside.

3. In another medium bowl, with an electric mixer at medium speed, whipped cream, sugar substitute, vanilla, and salt until stiff peaks form, about 4 min Fold the whipped cream into the cheese mixture in 3 additions.

4. Spread on cans, cover with fine gauze. Place the box on the rack above the baking sheet. Leave to cool for 12 to 24 hours or until solid. If desired, serve with mashed berries, sweetened with a sugar substitute.

Prep time:30 min; **Servings:** 4

Macros: 2.1 g net Carbs 3.3 g protein 16.4 g fat 0 g fiber 167.7 Cal

COFFEE PUNCH

Ingredients

- 2 large eggs (whole)

- 1 tsp sucralose sweetener (sugar substitute)

- ½ tsp vanilla extract

- 1 cup (8 fluid oz) of coffee (ground, decaffeinated)

- 1 cup heavy cream

- 4 fluid oz (without ice) Rum

- 1/8 cinnamon tsp

Instructions

5. In a small bowl, beat eggs and sugar substitute. Add vanilla, coffee, cream, and rum (if applicable); Mix well

6. Sprinkle the top with cinnamon.

Prep time:5 min; **Servings:** 1

Macros: 2.1 g net Carbs 4.4 g protein 24.5 g fat 0 g fiber 308.4 Cal

COFFEE FLAN WHIPPED CREAM

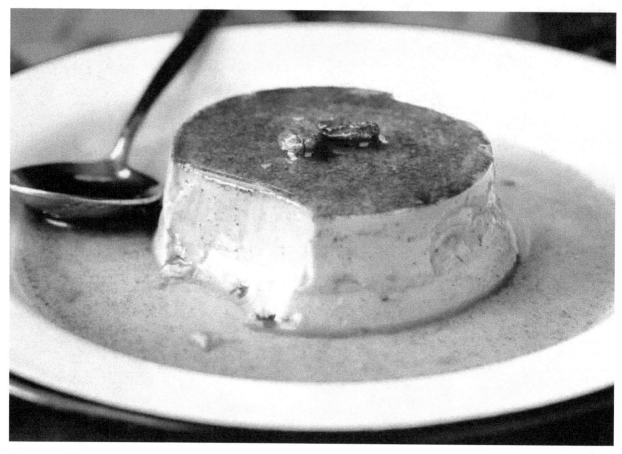

Ingredients

- 1 1/8 cup heavy cream

- 5 ¼ oz liquid espresso coffee

- 3 Tbsp sucralose sweetener (sugar substitute)

- 3 large eggs (whole)

- 4 Tbsp unsweetened flavored syrup - caramel

Instructions

1. Preheat the oven to 325° F.

2. Combine 1 cup cream, espresso, and sugar substitute in a medium-thick saucepan; Heat until small bubbles appear around the edge, about 3 min Beat the eggs in a medium bowl. Gradually add about a third of the hot cream mixture. Beat the egg mixture in the coffee mixture. Reduce the heat to low and cook, beating for 1 minute.

3. Pour into 4 6-oz molds or cups of cream (if the mixture looks lumpy, pour into a colander). Place the cups in a large roasting box. Place the roasting pan in the oven and carefully pour boiling water into the pan until the water reaches half the glasses. Cover the pan well with aluminum foil and make sure the paper does not touch the pastry cream and cook until the pastry cream is ready for about 35 min.

4. Remove from the oven and let stand for 10 min at room temperature. Remove the pastry cream from the roaster and dry; Cover with plastic wrap and stretch the aluminum foil so that it does not touch the pastry cream. Cold to cold, at least 3 hours.

5. Soak the cups halfway in boiling water for a few seconds; Glue a sharp knife along the edge to release it. Place a dessert plate on the cream and turn, shaking gently so as not to form. (Otherwise, serve the flakes in the cups.)

6. Place the caramel sauce in the microwave in a microwave bowl on high temperature to mix for about 10 seconds. Beat the remaining 1/8 cup cream. Caramel spray syrup on pies; Serve with whipped cream on the side and espresso beans to garnish, if desired.

Prep time: 20 min; **Servings:** 10

Macros: 3.2 g net Carbs 6.1 g protein 28.7 g fat 0 g fiber 291.6 Cal

BLUEBERRY CUSTARD

Ingredients

- 1 cup, whole blueberries

- 8 g of unsweetened French vanilla syrup

- ¼ cup vanilla whey protein (no added sugar)

- 3 cups of tap water

- 2 ½ sachets of jelly, sugar-free

- 4 individual packages of sucralose sweetener (sugar substitute)

Instructions

1. Mix in a blender of blueberries, vanilla syrup, and a smoothie. Puree until smooth.

2. For 1 cup cold water into a bowl, Sprinkle the jelly in water and let stand for 1 minute.

3. Mix the 2 remaining cups of water with a sugar substitute and cook (in the microwave or on the stove). Add the hot

water mixture to the gelatin mixture; Stir until gelatin dissolves.

4. Add the berry mixture and stir until smooth. For into 8 cups of custard. Let cool for at least 3 hours to set.

Prep time:20 min; **Servings:** 4

Macros: 1.6 g net Carbs 8.2 g protein 0 g fat 0.7 g fiber 41.9 Cal

CRANBERRY AND GINGERBREAD

Ingredients

- 1 ¼ cups whole wheat flour

- 3 tsp baking powder (straight phosphate, double effect)

- ½ cup peeled English walnuts (50 halves)

- 2 large Protein

- ¼ tsp salt

- ½ cup unsalted butter bar

- 2/3 cup sucralose sweetener (sugar substitute)

- 2 sour cream Tbsp (cultivated)

- 1 Tbsp ginger

- 1 tsp vanilla extract

- 1 cup, whole blueberries

- 2 large eggs (whole)

Instructions

4. Preheat to 350° F. Roast the nuts in an even layer on a baking sheet for 8 min. Let cool, place the nuts in a food processor until they are finely ground.

5. Grease a 9 x 5 x 3-inch loaf pan with spray oil.

6. Combine soy flour, baking powder, nuts, and salt in a large bowl. Beat in a medium bowl with an electric mixer on medium heat, butter, and sugar substitute until light, about 3 min.

7. In a medium bowl, beat the egg whites until firm but not dry, forming peaks. Gently fold egg whites into the dough until they meet. Place the dough in the prepared pan and bake for 40 to 45 min until a toothpick comes out clean.

8. Let cool in a pan on a rack for 10 min before removing. Bake the bread on a wire rack for at least 30 min before cutting it.

Prep time: 5 min **Servings:** 10

Macros: 2.9 g net Carbs 4 g protein 8.5 g fat 1.1 g fiber 104.7 Cal

BLUEBERRY AND RASPBERRY DESSERT

Ingredients

- 2 sachets of gelatin, sugar-free

- ½ cup tap water

- 2 cups (8 fluid oz) low-calorie cranberry juice with vitamin C

- 8 Tbsp unsweetened flavored syrup - Raspberry

- 2 tsp fresh lemon juice

Instructions

1. Put the jelly in a large bowl. Boil water. For water over the, stir until dissolved.

2. Add cranberry juice, raspberry syrup, and lemon juice. Mix well.

3. Divide the mixture among 6 dessert glasses. Cool up to 3 hours.

Prep time: 20 min; **Servings:** 6

Macros: 3.8 g net Carbs 2 g protein 0 g fat 0 g fiber 23.4 Cal.

CONCLUSION

We've come to the end of this trip, have you all baked?

I know at the beginning they may seem difficult to prepare but you just need to train a little bit, try and try again and you will see excellent results!

Dessert is always a meal very much appreciated by all, but that you can not always afford if you want to stay thin. Now you can.

I recommend everyone to always talk to a nutritionist before doing any diet, and enjoy the taste. Enjoy.

CPSIA information can be obtained
at www.ICGtesting.com
Printed in the USA
BVHW061225130421
604816BV00004B/918